Table of Contents

1

INTRODUCTION

A hiatal hernia is a condition in which a portion of the stomach protrudes through an opening in the diaphragm, the muscle that separates the abdomen from the chest. This can lead to a variety of unpleasant symptoms, including heartburn, acid reflux, difficulty swallowing, and chest pain. Managing a hiatal hernia often requires a multi-faceted approach, with dietary modifications playing a crucial role.

The hiatal hernia diet is designed to alleviate the symptoms associated with this condition and prevent further complications. The primary goals of this dietary approach are:

• **Reducing Acid Reflux:** By focusing on foods that are less likely to trigger acid reflux, the diet helps minimize the amount of stomach acid that flows back into the esophagus.

• **Promoting Healthy Digestion:** Certain dietary changes can improve the overall function of the digestive system, reducing the strain on the hiatal hernia.

• **Maintaining a Healthy Weight:** Excess weight can exacerbate the symptoms of a hiatal hernia, so the diet emphasizes foods that can help maintain a healthy body weight.

During the initial stages of managing a hiatal hernia, the diet may recommend a focus on low-fat, low-fiber, and low-residue foods. This can help reduce the burden on the digestive system and alleviate acute symptoms. **Examples of foods that may be included in this phase of the diet include:**

Lean proteins: Chicken, turkey, and fish

Refined grains: White bread, pasta, and rice

Cooked vegetables: Carrots, green beans, and squash

Certain fruits: Bananas, melons, and applesauce

Dairy products: Low-fat or non-fat milk, yogurt, and cheese

As the condition stabilizes and the individual's symptoms improve, the diet gradually transitions to a more balanced, fiber-rich approach. **This phase focuses on:**

Whole grains: Whole wheat, oats, quinoa, and brown rice

Fruits and vegetables: A variety of fresh, frozen, or canned produce, with an emphasis on those that are easy to digest

Lean proteins: Chicken, turkey, fish, and legumes

Healthy fats: Avocado, olive oil, and nuts (in moderation)

It's important to note that certain foods may exacerbate the symptoms of a hiatal hernia and should be limited or avoided, **such as:**

Spicy, fried, or fatty foods

Citrus fruits and juices

Tomatoes and tomato-based products

Caffeine (found in coffee, tea, and sodas)

Alcohol

Peppermint and chocolate

In addition to the dietary guidelines, the hiatal hernia diet also recommends:

Eating smaller, more frequent meals throughout the day to avoid overwhelming the digestive system

Avoiding lying down or exercising immediately after eating

Elevating the head of the bed during sleep to prevent acid reflux

Maintaining a healthy weight through a balanced diet and regular exercise

It's important to work closely with a healthcare provider or registered dietitian when following the hiatal hernia diet, as individual responses may vary. They can help you develop a personalized plan that takes into account your specific symptoms, dietary preferences, and any other underlying health conditions.

By adhering to the hiatal hernia diet and incorporating other lifestyle modifications, many individuals are able to effectively manage their condition, reduce the frequency and severity of symptoms, and improve their overall quality of life.

WHAT IS A HIATAL HERNIA?

A hiatal hernia occurs when the upper part of your stomach pushes up through your diaphragm and into your chest region.

The diaphragm is a large muscle that lies between your abdomen and chest. You use this muscle to help you breathe. Normally, your stomach is below the diaphragm, but in people with a hiatal hernia, a portion of the stomach pushes up through the muscle. The opening it moves through is called a hiatus.

Types of hiatal hernia

There are generally two types of hiatal hernia: sliding hiatal hernias and fixed, or paraesophageal, hernias.

Sliding hiatal hernia

This is the more prevalent form of hiatal hernia. It happens when your stomach and esophagus move into and out of your chest through the hiatus. Sliding hernias are typically small and often don't induce any symptoms, therefore may not necessitate treatment.

Fixed hiatal hernia

This hernia variant, less frequent and known as a paraesophageal hernia, involves a section of your stomach protruding through your diaphragm and staying in position. Although typically not severe, there's a possibility of blood flow to your stomach being blocked. Should this happen, it may lead to substantial harm and is considered a medical emergency.

Symptoms of a hiatal hernia

It's rare for even fixed hiatal hernias to cause symptoms. If you do experience any symptoms, they're usually caused by stomach acid, bile, or air entering your esophagus. Common symptoms include:

• heartburn that gets worse when you lean over or lie down

• acid reflux or GERD

• chest pain or epigastric pain

• trouble swallowing

• belching

Diet

Hiatal hernia causes acid reflux symptoms. Changing your diet can reduce your symptoms. It may help to eat smaller meals several times a day instead of three large meals. You should also avoid eating meals or snacks within a few hours of going to bed.

There are also certain foods that may increase your risk of heartburn. Consider avoiding:

• spicy foods

• chocolate

• foods made with tomatoes

• caffeine

• onions

• citrus fruits

• alcohol

Other ways to reduce your symptoms include:

• stopping smoking

• raising the head of your bed by at least 6 inches

• avoiding bending over or lying down after eating

Causes and risk factors for hiatal hernias

The precise cause of many hiatal hernias remains uncertain. For some individuals, injury or other forms of damage may weaken muscle tissue, allowing the stomach to push through the diaphragm. Another factor is exerting excessive pressure repeatedly on the muscles around the stomach. **This can happen when:**

• coughing

• vomiting

• straining during bowel movements

• lifting heavy objects

Some people are also born with an abnormally large hiatus. This makes it easier for the stomach to move through it.

Factors that can increase your risk of a hiatal hernia include:

• obesity

• aging

• smoking

You may not avoid a hiatal hernia entirely, but you can avoid making a hernia worse by:

• losing excess weight

• not straining during bowel movements

• getting help when lifting heavy objects

• avoiding tight belts and certain abdominal exercises

What is the connection between GERD and hiatal hernias?

Gastroesophageal reflux disease (GERD) occurs when the food, liquids, and acid in your stomach end up in your esophagus. This can lead to heartburn or nausea after meals. It's common for people with a hiatal hernia to have GERD. However, that doesn't mean either condition always causes the other. You can have a hiatal hernia without GERD or GERD without a hernia.

HIATAL HERNIA DIET

Hiatal hernias lead to symptoms of acid reflux. Adjusting your diet can alleviate these symptoms. Eating smaller, frequent meals throughout the day instead of three large ones and avoiding meals or snacks shortly before bedtime can be beneficial.

Opting for foods that are low in acid content can help alleviate this symptom.

Below, you'll find information on foods to avoid, foods to incorporate into your diet, and additional lifestyle recommendations for managing a hiatal hernia.

A hiatal hernia diet primarily focuses on minimizing symptoms of acid reflux and regurgitation by avoiding or limiting foods that relax the LES muscle or irritate the lining of the esophagus.

Foods and beverages to avoid

The foods and beverages you should avoid are the same ones you'd want to skip if you had gastroesophageal reflux disease (GERD).

These foods include:

• onions and garlic

• certain citrus fruits such as limes and oranges

• tomatoes and tomato-based foods, such as salsa and spaghetti sauce

• spicy foods

• fried foods

• foods high in sodium

• cocoa and chocolate

• peppermint and mint

Beverages to avoid include:

• alcohol, such as wine, beer, and spirits

• coffee

• caffeinated teas

• carbonated drinks, such as seltzer water and soda

• whole milk

However, depending on the severity of your hiatal hernia, these foods may or may not cause symptoms.

As such, you should keep a food journal so you can document which foods trigger your symptoms and avoid or limit them going forward.

It's also possible that you may still be able to tolerate these foods in small amounts so keeping a food diary can also help you identify the amounts of a food you can eat before it triggers symptoms.

Beyond avoiding or limiting the foods that may trigger symptoms, you should follow a varied, nutrient-dense diet consisting primarily of fruits, vegetables, whole grains, lean proteins, and healthy fats.

Foods and beverages to eat

There are still plenty of good foods that won't produce as much acid in your stomach. Many whole foods, for example, are good options because they aren't processed. This means they contain more fiber, which can help with acid reflux.

Try eating:

• non-citrus fruits, such as apples, pears, melons, and berries

• vegetables, such as artichokes, carrots, sweet potatoes, asparagus, squash, green beans, leafy greens, and peas

• whole grains

• nuts and seeds, like almonds and chia seeds

• lean protein

• yogurt

• plant-based milks, like soy or almond milk

• certain juices, like aloe vera, carrot, or cabbage juice

Hernia surgery repair diet

If you require hernia surgery there isn't necessarily a specific diet you have to follow post-hernia repair.

However, your surgeon may recommend that you temporarily follow a dysphagia diet since many people experience difficulty swallowing after surgery.

With a dysphagia diet, the consistency of your drinks, food, or both are modified to promote safe and efficient swallowing.

Most people who receive hernia repair surgery experience few or no symptoms but recurrent hiatal hernias are still possible, especially in those with larger hernias.

Diet likely has no significant role in preventing the recurrence of a hiatal hernia but you should still follow a varied, nutrient-dense diet to support overall health and reduce further harm to your esophagus that may have been caused by the hiatal hernia.

3-day sample hiatal hernia diet

Here's a 3-day sample hiatal hernia diet that excludes common foods that may trigger heartburn and regurgitation:

Day 1

- Breakfast: cottage cheese toast with avocado

- Lunch: grilled chicken wrap

- Snack: Greek yogurt and walnuts

- Dinner: roasted pork loin, carrots, and brussels sprouts

Day 2 (vegan option)

- Breakfast: high-fiber cereal topped with soymilk and berries

- Lunch: chickpea salad

- Snack: apple slices and almonds

• Dinner: Mediterranean quinoa pasta salad

Day 3

• Breakfast: spinach and eggs scramble and oatmeal topped with fruit

• Lunch: grilled lemon chicken salad

• Snack: string cheese stick, strawberries, and almonds

• Dinner: roasted salmon and green beans with brown rice

Eating and cooking tips

Even the way you cook and eat your foods can make a difference. People who experience heartburn should try to prepare their foods in healthy ways. For example, fried foods can trigger heartburn. Also, eating too much at one time may also make your symptoms worse.

Some tips:

• Cook with healthy fats, like avocado, coconut, and olive oils.

• Eat whole foods whenever possible. The fiber content of these foods should help with your acid reflux. Also, the less processed the food is, the better.

• Eat small meals every few hours instead of three large meals during the day.

• Add probiotic foods to your diet. Cultured vegetables, like pickles, are a tasty option. Yogurt, kefir, and kombucha are other good choices. Taking a probiotic supplement is also an option.

• Drink plain water. It's the best beverage you can drink. You should aim to drink eight glasses of water per day. Try adding lemon to your water for additional acid-lowering power. Lemon is a fruit that, although acidic outside the body, is metabolized to have alkaline byproducts.

Other lifestyle tips

Beyond food, there are many things you can do to help prevent and deal with acid reflux from your hiatal hernia:

• Don't lie down after eating. Try to wait at least two or three hours before going to bed after dinner.

• You may want to elevate the head of your bed about 6 inches in order to sleep more comfortably.

• Work with your doctor to reach a healthy weight if you're overweight.

• Skip tight-fitting clothes, which can make your heartburn worse.

• Ask your doctor about over-the-counter (OTC) or prescription medications that may reduce the acid in your stomach. Some OTC suggestions include probiotics and digestive enzymes.

• Eat in a calm and relaxing place. Avoid standing up while eating.

HIATAL HERNIA DIET COOKBOOK

Chilled Pea Soup with Herbs

Ingredients

• 1 Tbsp olive oil

• 2 medium white onions (sliced)

- 2 cups low sodium chicken or vegetable broth

- 1 lb frozen peas

- 2 cups fresh spinach

- 1/4 tsp salt

- fresh ground black pepper (to taste)

- 1 Tbsp fresh tarragon

- 2 Tbsp fresh parsley

- 1/4 cup fresh chives

- 1/4 cup fresh mint

- 3 ounces semi-soft goat cheese

Direction

- Prepare a large mixing bowl filled with ice. The bowl should be large enough for the sauce pan to fit into and be surrounded by ice.

- Place the olive oil in a large sauce pan over medium-high heat. When hot add the onions. Cook, stirring almost continuously, for about 8 minutes until the onions are translucent. Do not let the onions brown.

• Add the chicken stock and increase the heat to high. Add the frozen peas.

• Stir occasionally. When the soup begins to come to a boil reduce the heat slightly so that it continues to simmer.

• Cook for about 5- 7 minutes, stirring frequently.

• Add the spinach and cook for another two minutes. Remove from the heat and add one cup of crushed ice.

• Place the pan in the ice bowl and stir until the ice in the soup melts. When the soup is slightly cool add the salt, pepper, tarragon, parley, chives, mint and goat cheese.

• Using a stick blender, or transferring to a blender in two batches, puree until smooth. Chill and serve.

Chilled Watermelon Soup

Ingredients

• 4 cups watermelon (seeded)

- 1 lb tomatoes (seeded)

- 2 Tbsp fresh lime juice

- 1/4 cup red bell pepper (diced)

- 1/4 tsp salt

- fresh ground black pepper (to taste)

- 4 tsp olive oil

- 8 leaves fresh basil (chiffonade)

Direction

- Place the watermelon, tomatoes, lime juice, red pepper, salt and pepper in a blender. Puree.

- Pour the soup into a tall pitcher. Place in the freezer. As the soup cools it will form two layers. At the top will be a thicker, dark red soup and below that a clearer watery liquid.

- Using a small measuring cup or a turkey baster, gently remove as much of the darker, thicker soup as you can and discard the watery liquid.

• Serve well chilled and topped with 1 teaspoon of olive oil (flavored oil works great) and the basil.

Classic Potato Soup

Ingredients

- 1 tsp olive or canola oil

- 1 large white onion (diced)

- 2 lbs Idaho potatoes (cut into 1 inch cubes)

- 5 cups water

- 1/2 cup 2% milk

- 1/4 tsp salt

- fresh ground black pepper (to taste)

- 4 ounces reduced fat cheddar cheese (shredded)

- green onion (sliced crosswise)

Direction

• Place the oil in a large saucepan over medium heat. Add the diced onion and cook, stirring frequently, for about 3 minutes.

• Add the potatoes and stir. Add the 5 cups of water and stir.

• Increase the heat until the water begins to boil and then reduce to medium-low so that the soup is simmering. Cook, stirring occasionally, for about 20 minutes until the potatoes are soft.

• Turn off the heat and let the soup cool slightly. Allow it to stand for about 5 minutes and then stir in the milk, salt and pepper.

• When ready to serve reheat the soup gently. Serve in bowls garnished with 1 ounce of cheddar cheese per serving and sprinkle with green onions.

Beef Stew

Ingredients

• 4 cups water

• 25 pearl onions (peeled)

- 1/3 cup all purpose white flour

- 1 tsp salt

- 1/4 tsp fresh ground black pepper

- 1 1/2 lbs flank steak (3/4 inch cubes)

- cooking spray

- 1/2 lb button mushrooms (quartered)

- 1 cup white onion (sliced)

- 1 Tbsp fresh lemon juice

- 1 Tbsp Worcestershire sauce

- 1 lb carrots (peeled and sliced 1/4 inch thick)

- 2 bay leaves

- 1 1/2 lbs red potatoes (peeled and 3/4 inch cubes)

- 1/8 tsp ground allspice

- 4 cups water

Methods

• Heat water in a medium stock-pot over high heat until it is at a shiver. Add pearl onions and cook for about ten minutes. Drain and place the onions in a large stock pot.

• Preheat oven to 400°F.

• Mix flour, salt and pepper in a paper bag. Toss the cubes of flank steak in the flour, coating well.

• Coat a large skillet with cooking spray and heat over medium-high heat. Add cubes of flank steak and cook, turning until all sides are brown. Do not overcrowd the beef or the meat will steam and not brown. Remove the meat to the stock pot as it browns.

• Add the onions to the skillet and cook until they are soft and brown. Add them to the stock pot.

• Add the lemon juice and Worcestershire sauce to the skillet and deglaze the pan, scraping up anything stuck to the bottom of the pan. Add the deglazing liquid to the stock pot.

• Add carrots, bay leaves, potatoes, allspice and water to the stock-pot.

- Place covered pot in the oven and reduce heat to 400°F.

- Cook for one hour stirring gently every fifteen minutes.

Borscht

Ingredients

- 2 lb beets

- 2 tsp olive oil

- 1 large white onion (diced)

- 5 cups water

- 1/2 lemon (juiced)

- 1/2 tsp salt

- fresh ground black pepper (to taste)

- 8 Tbsp reduced fat sour cream

- 16 tsp fresh dill

Direction

• Wash the beets well. Wrap in aluminum foil. Place in the oven and set the temperature to 325°F. Roast for 60 minutes. Remove and let cool. Peel the beets and set aside 1/2 pound.

• Place the olive oil a large sauce pan over medium high heat. Add the onion and cook for about 5 minutes, stirring frequently. Chop the remaining 1 1/2 pound of peeled beets into large dice. Add to the pan with the onions. Add the water, lemon juice, salt and pepper. Cover, and when the soup begins to boil, reduce the heat to medium low so that it is simmering.

• Cook for about 60 minutes, stirring occasionally.

• While the soup is cooking, dice the remaining beets into 1/3 inch cubes. Chill.

• When the soup is done, let it cool and then puree smooth. Add the cubed beets and chill the soup.

• When ready to serve, ladle the soup into bowls and top each serving with a tablespoon of sour cream and a 2 teaspoons of fresh dill.

• Using a potato peeler, peel the stems to expose the tender center.

• Dice the peeled stems.

• Place them in a stock-pot with the four cups of water on medium heat and simmer until tender.

• This will take about 20 minutes and the water will be reduced by about half. When they are soft, drain and add to the ice water.

• While the stems are boiling, steam the flowerets until they are bright green and slightly tender: about 8-10 minutes.

• When they are cooked, plunge them into ice water to stop them from cooking further.

• After they are cool, chop finely.

• After the stems are soft, using a blender or stick blender, puree them and the water they cooked in until smooth.

• Place the olive oil in a medium stock-pot over medium-high heat and add the onions.

• Cook the onions slowly, stirring almost continuously, until soft and they are well caramelized. This should take about 20 minutes.

• Add the flour and stir until well blended.

31

- Add the milk and stir.

- Add the pureed broccoli stems, half of the broccoli flowerets, and salt.

- As the soup thickens, blend it smooth using a blender or stick blender.

- Finely chop the remaining broccoli flowerets and stir into the soup.

- As the soup reheats, add the cheese in 3 batches and allow it to melt.

- Heat gently on low for about 5 minutes and serve.

Butternut Squash Soup

Ingredients

- 2 cups water

- 2 lbs butternut squash

- 1/2 tsp salt

- fresh ground black pepper

- 1/2 tsp dried thyme leaves

- 1/8 tsp ground nutmeg

- 1 cup water

Direction

- Place the water in a large sauce pan fitted with a steamer basket over high heat. Put the cubed squash in the steamer basket. Steam until tender (20 - 30 minutes).

- Let the squash cool and then add it to the remaining steaming water in the bottom of the sauce pan. Using a stick blender or a blender puree the squash and water until smooth.

- Place the pan over low heat and add the salt, pepper, thyme leaves and ground nutmeg.

- Reheat the soup gently. Stir in the remaining water to the desired consistency. It may take as much as 1 1/2 to 2 cups.

Cannellini Bean Soup

Ingredients

• 2 1/3 cups cannellini beans (or 2 15-ounce cans no salt added cannellini beans)

• 3 quarts water

• 1 tsp olive oil

• 2 cloves garlic (minced)

• 1 large white onion (diced)

• 2 cups low sodium chicken or vegetable broth

• 1/4 tsp salt

• 2 ribs celery with leaves (minced)

• 2 Tbsp fresh oregano

• fresh ground black pepper

Direction

• Place the beans in a large pot and cover with water. Let the beans soak overnight. Drain the beans the next day and cover with water, then place over medium-high heat. Bring to a boil and reduce the heat to a simmer. Let the beans cook for about an hour until soft.

• Drain the beans and set aside. Rinse the pot well. (Alternatively use 2 - 15 ounce cans no salt added cannellini beans.)

• Place the olive oil in the same pot over medium heat. Add the garlic and white onion. Cook slowly over medium until the onions are translucent. Add the beans back to the pot and stir well.

• Add the chicken stock and salt. Cook for about 10 minutes stirring occasionally. Add the celery, fresh oregano and black pepper. Cook for about 20 minutes.

• Using a stick blender (or a conventional blender in batches), blend the soup until it is pureed. The soup may be served hot or chilled.

Chicken and Black-Eyed Pea Soup

Ingredients

- 1 tsp olive oil

- 1 large red onion (diced)

- 2 ribs celery (diced)

- 1 lb boneless skinless chicken thighs (cut into 1 inch cubes)

- 2 tsp dried sage

- 1/2 tsp dried thyme

- 1/2 tsp salt

- fresh ground black pepper to taste

- 3 cups low sodium chicken or vegetable broth

- 2 cups water

- 2 15-ounce cans no salt added black eyed peas (drained and rinsed)

- 8 ounces fresh spinach

Directon

• Place the olive oil in a large sauce pan over medium heat. Add the red onion and celery and cook, stirring frequently, for about 5 - 7 minutes until the onions begin to soften.

• Add the chicken thighs, sage and thyme and cook, stirring frequently, until the chicken is lightly browned - about 5 - 7 minutes.

• Add the salt, pepper, chicken stock, water and black eyed peas. Increase the heat to high and when the soup begins to boil reduce the heat to medium or medium-low so that the soup simmers.

• Cook for about 40 minutes, stirring occasionally.

• When ready to serve, place 2 ounces of spinach in the bottom of a bowl and top with two cups of soup.

BREAKFAST RECIPES

Breads and Muffins

Apple Cinnamon Bread

Ingredients

- 1/4 cup pecans (coarsely chopped)

- 2 tsp maple syrup

- 1/4 tsp ground cinnamon

- 1 large egg yolk

- 1 tsp canola oil

- 2/3 cup Z-Sweet stevia or Splenda

- 1/2 cup unsweetened applesauce

- 1/2 tsp pure vanilla extract

- 3 large egg whites

- 1 1/4 cups all purpose white flour

- 3/4 cup whole wheat flour

- 1/4 tsp salt

- 2 tsp baking powder

- 1/2 tsp baking soda

- 1 tsp ground cinnamon

- 1/4 cup wheat germ

- 2 cups apples (peeled and grated)

- 1/2 cup low-fat buttermilk

Direction

- Preheat oven to 350°F. Line a 1 1/2 quart glass Pyrex oblong loaf pan with foil (non-stick foil works best).

- Combine the pecans, maple syrup and cinnamon in a small bowl. Stir until well blended. Set aside.

- Whisk the egg yolk until smooth. Add the canola oil and whisk together until smooth. Add the Z-Sweet or Splenda, applesauce and vanilla extract and whisk until smooth.

- In separate bowl whisk the egg whites until they begin to be very frothy and white. Do not beat into stiff peaks.

• Place the all-purpose flour, whole wheat flour, salt, baking powder, baking soda, cinnamon and wheat germ in a sifter and sift into the mixing bowl.

• Gently fold the creamed mixture together with the flour mixture. As this is blended add the grated apples.

• Just as the apples are blended in add buttermilk and fold until smooth. As soon as the mixture is well blended add the frothed egg whites and fold together until smooth.

• Pour the batter into the lined Pyrex dish. Spread the pecan and maple syrup mixture evenly over the top and place in the preheated oven. Bake for 60 minutes.

Banana Nut Bread

Ingredients

• 1 large egg yolk

• 1 tsp canola oil

• 2/3 cup Z-Sweet stevia or Splenda

• 1/2 tsp pure vanilla extract

- 2 medium bananas

- 3 large egg whites

- 1 1/4 cup all purpose white flour

- 3/4 cup whole wheat flour

- 1/4 tsp salt

- 2 tsp baking powder

- 1/2 tsp baking soda

- 1/2 tsp ground cinnamon

- 1/4 tsp ground nutmeg

- 1/4 cup wheat germ

- 1/2 cup pecans (coarsely chopped)

- 1/4 cup low-fat buttermilk

- 2 tsp light brown sugar

Direction

- Preheat oven to 350°F. Line a 1 1/2 quart glass Pyrex oblong loaf pan with foil (non-stick foil works best).

- Whisk the egg yolk until smooth. Add the canola oil and whisk together until smooth.

- Using the whisk, mash the bananas into the mixture until smooth. Add the Z-Sweet or Splenda and vanilla extract and whisk until smooth.

- In separate bowl whisk the egg whites until they begin to be very frothy and white. Do not beat into stiff peaks.

- Place the all-purpose flour, whole wheat flour, salt, baking powder, baking soda, cinnamon, nutmeg and wheat germ in a sifter and sift into the mixing bowl.

- Gently fold the creamed mixture together with the flour mixture. As this is blended add the pecans. As soon as the mixture is well blended add the frothed egg whites and fold together until smooth.

- Just as the pecans are blended in, add buttermilk and fold until smooth.

• Pour the batter into the lined Pyrex dish and sprinkle the light brown sugar evenly over the top. Place the loaf pan in the preheated oven. Bake for 55 minutes.

Banana Nut Muffins

Ingredients

• 1 large egg (separated)

• 2 tsp unsalted butter

• 1 large banana

• 1/2 tsp pure vanilla extract

• 1/2 cup Z-Sweet stevia or Splenda

• 1/4 cup chopped pecans

• 1 cup all purpose white flour

• 1/2 cup whole wheat flour

• 2 Tbsp wheat germ

• 1/4 tsp salt

• 1 tsp baking powder

43

- 1/4 tsp baking soda

- 1/2 tsp ground cinnamon

- 1/4 tsp ground nutmeg

- 1/4 cup low-fat buttermilk

- 2 tsp light brown sugar

Direction

- Preheat oven to 375°F.

- Using a whisk, cream together the egg yolk and light spread. Add the banana and mash into the mixture until well blended. Add the vanilla extract and Splenda and blend. Fold in the chopped pecans.

- Sift the all purpose flour, whole wheat flour, wheat germ, salt, baking powder, baking soda, cinnamon and nutmeg in a sifter and sift into the mixing bowl.

- Gently fold the creamed mixture together with the flour mixture until smooth. When blended the mixture will still be dry. Whisk the egg white until it is white and foamy (about tripled in volume). Fold in the egg white.

• Fold in the buttermilk, and when the dough is just blended together, stop.

• Line a standard size muffin tin with 6 muffin papers and fill each muffin paper with an equal amount of batter. Sprinkle the brown sugar over the tops of the muffins.

• Place the muffins in the oven and bake for 20 minutes.

Blueberry Muffins

Ingredients

• 1 large egg

• 2 Tbsp. reduced-fat spread

• 1/2 cup Splenda or stevia

• 2 Tbsp. non-fat yogurt

• 1/2 tsp. pure vanilla extract

• 1 cup all purpose flour

- 1/2 cup whole wheat flour

- 2 Tbsp. wheat germ

- 1/4 tsp. salt

- 1 tsp. baking powder

- 1/4 tsp. baking soda

- 1/2 cup low-fat buttermilk

- 1/2 cup blueberries

Direction

• Separate the egg into an egg white and egg yolk. Set the egg yolk aside and whisk the egg white until frothy. Add the reduced-fat spread and whisk together until smooth. Add the Splenda®, egg yolk, yogurt and vanilla extract.

• Whisk until smooth.

• Place the all-purpose flour, whole wheat flour, wheat germ, salt, baking powder and baking soda in a sifter and sift into the mixing bowl.

• Gently fold the creamed mixture together with the flour mixture. As this is blended slowly add the buttermilk folding until smooth. As soon as the mixture is well blended, stop.

• Gently fold the blueberries into the batter. Do not over mix.

• Line a muffin tin with 6 muffin papers and fill each muffin paper with an equal amount of batter. Bake for 12 – 15 minutes.

Raisin Bran Muffins

Ingredients

• 1 1/2 cups Fiber One Bran Cereal

• 1/2 cup 2% milk

• 1/4 cup low-fat buttermilk

• 1 large egg yolk

• 1 Tbsp unsalted butter

• 1/2 cup unsweetened applesauce

• 1/2 cup Splenda or stevia

- 2/3 cup all purpose flour

- 2/3 cup whole wheat flour

- 1 tsp baking powder

- 1/4 tsp baking soda

- 1/4 tsp salt

- 1/2 tsp ground nutmeg

- 3 large egg whites

- 1 cup seedless raisins

Direction

- Place the bran cereal, milk and buttermilk in a mixing bowl. Let the mixture stand for about 20 minutes until the bran is softened. Using a whisk mash the bran until it is well blended into the milk and forms a paste. There will be some larger pieces. This is OK.

- Preheat oven to 375°F.

• Cream together the egg yolk and butter until smooth. Add the applesauce and the Z-Sweet or Splenda and whisk until smooth.

• Sift the all-purpose flour, whole wheat flour, baking powder, baking soda, salt and nutmeg into the mixing bowl.

• Sprinkle the raisins over the top of the flour mixture and then fold the flour and raisin mixture together with the bran mixture.

• Whisk the egg whites until white and frothy (they should about triple in volume). Fold the egg whites into the muffin mixture until they are just blended in.

• Line a standard size muffin tin with 6 muffin papers and fill each muffin paper with an equal amount of batter. Bake for 20 - 25 minutes.

Cornbread Muffins

Ingredients

• 3/4 cup yellow cornmeal

• 1 cup all purpose flour

- 1/3 cup sugar

- 1 Tbsp baking powder

- 1/2 tsp salt

- 1 cup non-fat buttermilk

- 1 large egg

- 1 Tbsp unsalted butter

Direction

- Mix all ingredients together in a bowl. Let stand for five to ten minutes.

- Line a non-stick muffin tin with muffin papers. Divide the batter into twelve muffins and bake at 325°F for about 15 minutes until golden on top.

Carrot Muffins

Ingredients

- 1 large egg (separated)

- 2 tsp canola oil

- 1/2 cup Z-Sweet stevia or Splenda

- 2 Tbsp non-fat yogurt

- 1/2 tsp pure vanilla extract

- 1 cup all purpose white flour

- 1/2 cup whole wheat flour

- 1/4 tsp salt

- 1 tsp baking powder

- 1/4 tsp baking soda

- 1/2 tsp ground cinnamon

- 1/4 tsp ground nutmeg

- 1 cup carrots (peeled and shredded)

- 1/4 cup oatmeal (quick, not instant)

- 1/2 cup low-fat buttermilk

Direction

• Preheat oven to 375°F.

• Separate the egg into an egg white and egg yolk. Set the egg yolk aside and whisk the egg white until frothy. Add the canola oil and whisk together until smooth. Add the Z-Sweet or Splenda®, egg yolk, yogurt and vanilla extract.

• Whisk until smooth.

• Place the all-purpose flour, whole wheat flour, salt, baking powder, baking soda, cinnamon and nutmeg in a sifter and sift into the mixing bowl. Sprinkle the flakes of oatmeal over the top.

• Gently fold the creamed mixture together with the flour and oatmeal mixture. As this is blended slowly add the shredded carrots.

• Just as the carrots are blended in add buttermilk until smooth. As soon as the mixture is well blended, stop.

• Line a muffin tin with muffin papers and fill each muffin paper with an equal amount of batter. Bake for 12 - 15 minutes.

Apple salad with figs and almonds

Ingredients

- 2 large red apples, cored and diced (about 4 cups)

- 6 dried figs, chopped (about 1 cup)

- 2 carrots, peeled and grated (about 3/4 cup)

- 2 ribs of celery, diced (about 2 cups)

- 1/2 cup fat-free lemon yogurt

- 2 tablespoons slivered almonds

Directions

- In a small bowl, combine apples, figs, carrots and celery. Add yogurt and mix thoroughly. Top with slivered almonds and serve.

Artichokes alla Romana

Ingredients

- 2 cups fresh breadcrumbs, preferably whole-wheat

• 1 tablespoon olive oil

• 4 large globe artichokes

• 2 lemons, halved

• 1/3 cup grated Parmesan cheese

• 3 garlic cloves, finely chopped

• 2 tablespoons finely chopped fresh flat-leaf (Italian) parsley

• 1 tablespoon grated lemon zest

• 1/4 teaspoon freshly ground black pepper

• 1 cup plus 2 to 4 tablespoons low-sodium vegetable or chicken stock

• 1 cup dry white wine

• 1 tablespoon minced shallot

• 1 teaspoon chopped fresh oregano

Directions

• Heat the oven to 400 F. In a bowl, combine the breadcrumbs and olive oil. Toss to coat. Spread the crumbs in a shallow baking pan and bake, stirring once halfway through, until the crumbs are lightly golden, about 10 minutes. Set aside to cool.

• Working with 1 artichoke at a time, snap off any tough outer leaves and trim the stem flush with the base. Cut off the top third of the leaves with a serrated knife, and trim off any remaining thorns with scissors. Rub the cut edges with a lemon half to prevent discoloration. Separate the inner leaves and pull out the small leaves from the center. Using a melon baller or spoon, scoop out the fuzzy choke, then squeeze some lemon juice into the cavity. Trim the remaining artichokes in the same manner.

• In a large bowl, toss the breadcrumbs with the Parmesan, garlic, parsley, lemon zest and pepper. Add the 2 to 4 tablespoons stock, 1 tablespoon at a time, using just enough for the stuffing to begin to stick together in small clumps.

• Using 2/3 of the stuffing, mound it slightly in the center of the artichokes. Then, starting at the bottom, spread the leaves open and spoon a rounded teaspoon of stuffing near the base of each leaf. (The artichokes can be prepared to this point several hours ahead and kept refrigerated.)

• In a Dutch oven with a tightfitting lid, combine the 1 cup stock, wine, shallot and oregano. (Note: Don't use cast iron or the cooked artichokes will turn brown.) Bring to a boil, then reduce the heat to low. Arrange the artichokes, stem-end down, in the liquid in a single layer. Cover and simmer until the outer leaves are tender, about 45 minutes (add water if necessary). Transfer the artichokes to a rack and let cool slightly. Cut each artichoke into quarters and serve warm.

Baby beet and orange salad

Ingredients

• 2 bunches baby beets with greens (about 4 cups of beets, 1 cup greens)

• 2 ribs celery, chopped (1/2 cup)

• 1/4 head Napa cabbage, chopped (1 1/2 cups)

• 1 small yellow onion, chopped (1/2 cup)

• Juice and zest of 1 orange

• 1 orange, peeled and cut into segments

- 1/2 tablespoon olive oil

- Black pepper to taste

Directions

- Heat oven to 400 F. Cut greens off of beets. Rinse greens under cold running water, drain well and reserve.

- Wash beets. Drizzle a bit of olive oil onto your hands and rub beets to coat them lightly. Wrap beets in foil and bake for about 45 minutes or until tender. Cool until you can handle and then pull off the outer skin. Slice and set aside.

- Cut beet greens into strips and place in mixing bowl. Chop celery, cabbage and onion, and add to bowl. Zest and juice 1 orange into bowl. Peel the other orange and cut into segments. Add to bowl. Drizzle 1/2 tablespoon olive oil over the salad. Season with black pepper and toss to combine.

- Arrange salad on chilled plates and top with sliced beets. Serve immediately.

Blue cheese, walnut spinach salad

Ingredients

Dressing:

• 4 teaspoons olive oil

• 2 tablespoons balsamic vinegar

• 1 tablespoon maple syrup

• 1/4 teaspoon nutmeg

• 1 tablespoon plain low-fat yogurt

Salad:

• 2 pounds spinach, roughly chopped (or 3 10-ounce packages)

• 1/2 cup sliced red onion

• 1 1/2 cups sliced cucumbers

• 1 1/2 cups grape tomatoes

• 1/4 cup chopped walnuts

• 1/4 cup blue cheese crumbles

Directions

• Combine ingredients for dressing in a blender or processor. Chill.

• Toss spinach greens with dressing and mound a generous 2 cups onto chilled plates.

• Layer vegetables, walnuts and blue cheese crumbles on top of spinach. Serve.

Braised celery root

Ingredients

• 1 cup vegetable stock or broth

• 1 celery root (celeriac), peeled and diced (about 3 cups)

• 1/4 cup sour cream

• 1 teaspoon Dijon mustard

• 1/4 teaspoon salt

• 1/4 teaspoon freshly ground black pepper

• 2 teaspoons fresh thyme leaves

Directions

• In a large saucepan, bring the stock to a boil over high heat. Stir in the celery root. When the stock returns to a boil, reduce the heat to low. Cover and simmer, stirring occasionally, until the celery root is tender, 10 to 12 minutes.

• Using a slotted spoon, transfer the celery root to a bowl, cover and keep warm. Raise the heat under the saucepan to high and bring the cooking liquid to a boil. Cook, uncovered, until reduced to 1 tablespoon, about 5 minutes.

• Remove from the heat and whisk in the sour cream, mustard, salt and pepper. Add the celery root and thyme to the sauce and stir over medium heat until heated through. Transfer to a warmed serving dish and serve immediately.

Butternut squash and apple salad

Ingredients

- 1 butternut squash, peeled and seeded, cut into 1/2-inch pieces (about 8 cups)

- 2 teaspoons olive oil

- 2 large apples, cored and cut 1/2-inch pieces

- 6 cups spinach, chopped

- 1 1/2 cups chopped celery

- 6 cups arugula, chopped

- 2 cups chopped carrots

Dressing:

- 1/2 cup low-fat plain yogurt

- 2 teaspoons balsamic vinegar

- 1 1/2 teaspoons honey

Directions

- Heat the oven to 400 F.

• Toss squash in olive oil, roast in oven for 20 to 30 minutes until golden brown and soft. Cool completely.

• Combine all vegetables in large bowl.

• Prepare dressing by mixing together yogurt, vinegar and honey. Whisk until smooth.

• Pour dressing over salad. Toss and enjoy.

Couscous salad

Ingredients

• 1 cup whole-wheat couscous

• 1 cup zucchini, cut into 1/4-inch pieces

• 1 medium red bell pepper, cut into 1/4-inch pieces

• 1/2 cup finely chopped red onion

• 3/4 teaspoon ground cumin

• 1/2 teaspoon ground black pepper

• 2 tablespoons extra virgin olive oil

• 1 tablespoon lemon juice

• Chopped fresh parsley, basil or oregano for garnish (optional)

Directions

• Cook couscous according to preparation instructions on the package.

• When couscous is cooked, fluff with fork. Mix in zucchini, bell pepper, onion, cumin and black pepper. Set aside.

• In a small bowl, whisk together the olive oil and lemon juice. Pour over the couscous mixture and toss to combine. Cover and refrigerate. Serve chilled. Garnish with fresh herbs.

Crab salad

Ingredients

• 1/4 cup lime juice

• 1/4 cup rice wine vinegar

• 1 teaspoon sugar

• 1 cucumber, seeded and thinly sliced

- 1/3 cup chopped fresh mint

- 12 ounces cooked crab meat, drained

- 4 cups mixed salad greens (mesclun) or romaine lettuce

- 4 lime wedges

Directions

- In a small bowl, combine the lime juice, vinegar, sugar, cucumber and mint. Add the crab and toss to coat well. Divide the lettuce among individual plates. Top with the crab mixture. Spoon any remaining dressing over the crab. Garnish with lime wedges and serve immediately

Cucumber pineapple salad

Ingredients

- 1/4 cup sugar

- 2/3 cup rice wine vinegar

- 2 tablespoons water

- 1 cup canned no-sugar added pineapple chunks

- 1 cucumber, peeled and thinly sliced

- 1 carrot, peeled and cut into thin strips

- 1/3 cup thinly sliced red onion

- 4 cups torn salad greens

- 1 tablespoon sesame seeds, toasted

Directions

- In a heavy saucepan, bring the sugar, vinegar and water to a boil. Stir constantly until reduced to about 1/2 cup, about 5 minutes. Transfer to a large bowl and place in the refrigerator until cool. Add the pineapple, cucumber, carrot and red onion to the mixture. Toss well.

- To serve, divide the salad greens among individual plates. Top with the pineapple mixture and sprinkle with toasted sesame seeds. Serve immediately.

Dilled shrimp salad on lettuce leaves

Ingredients

• 2 cups uncooked farfalle (bow tie) pasta

• 4 fresh asparagus stalks, cut into 1/2-inch pieces

• 1/4 cup reduced-sodium or light vinaigrette salad dressing

• 1 1/2 teaspoons fresh dill

• 1/2 pound cooked shrimp

• 8 cherry tomatoes, halved

• 4 scallions or green onions, diced

• 4 cups watercress or another type of salad greens

Directions

• Fill a large pot 3/4 full with water and bring to a boil. Add the pasta and cook until al dente (tender), 10 to 12 minutes, or according to the package directions. Drain the pasta thoroughly and rinse under cold water.

• In a small saucepan, cover the asparagus with water. Bring to a boil and cook only until tender-crisp, about 3 to 5 minutes. Drain and rinse under cold water. In a small bowl, add the salad dressing and dill. Whisk to mix evenly.

• In a large bowl, add the pasta, asparagus, shrimp, tomatoes and scallions. Add the salad dressing mixture and toss to coat evenly. Cover and refrigerate until thoroughly chilled, about 1 hour.

• To serve, divide the watercress among the plates. Top with dilled salad and serve.

SIDES

Artichoke and Spinach Dip

Ingredients

• 2 15-ounce cans artichoke hearts (packed in water)

• 2 10-ounce packages frozen spinach (thawed)

• 1/2 cup fat-free mayonnaise

• 2 1/2 ounces mozzarella cheese (grated)

• 1 ounce reduced-fat cream cheese

• 1/4 tsp salt

• 1/8 tsp ground nutmeg

Direction

• After the spinach has thawed, drain it well, pressing all of the liquid out through a sieve into a bowl. Do not discard the liquid as you will use some of this liquid later.

• Drain the artichoke hearts and place them in a food processor. Add the spinach, mozzarella, cream cheese, salt, nutmeg and mayonnaise. Process until almost smooth. Add some of the spinach liquid, 1 Tablespoon at a time, to help achieve that smoothness. One to two Tablespoons is usually enough.

• When ready to serve, place the dip in a microwave-safe bowl. Put the dip in the microwave and heat in 30 second intervals, stirring well in between each 30 second interval. The dip should be hot enough to let the cheese melt and add to the creaminess of the dip, but not too hot or you will overcook the spinach. Serve immediately.

Artichoke Dip

Ingredients

- 2 15 ounce can artichoke hearts (packed in water)

- 1/4 cup fat free mayonnaise

- 2 ounces mozzarella cheese (grated)

- 1/4 tsp dried tarragon

- fresh ground black pepper (to taste)

Direction

- Drain the artichoke hearts and place in a food processor. Process for about 5 seconds.

- Add the mayonnaise, mozzarella, tarragon and pepper. Process until almost smooth.

• When ready to serve place the dip in a glass dish. Put the dish in the microwave and heat in 30 second intervals, stirring well.

Baked Tortilla Chips

Ingredients

• 2 corn tortillas

• spray oil (olive or canola oil)

• 1/4 tsp salt

• fresh ground black pepper or other spice of your choice to taste

Direction

• Preheat oven to 400F.

• Cut each tortilla into 8 pie-shaped slices and spread onto baking sheets in a single layer.

• Lightly spray both sides with cooking oil.

• Sprinkle the salt over the tortilla slices and add pepper (or your spice of choice) to taste.

• Bake for 10 to 14 minutes or until chips start to turn light brown.

Candied Pecans

Ingredients

• 1/2 cup pecan pieces

• 1/16 tsp salt

• 2 tsp maple syrup

Direction

• Place a sheet of wax paper on the kitchen counter.

• Place the pecans in a non-stick skillet over medium-high heat. Cook, stirring frequently, for about 5 minutes. Watch the nuts closely and as they begin to brown reduce the heat to medium.

• Add the salt. Cook for about one minute more until the pecans are browned.

• Add the maple syrup and let it bubble for about ten seconds shaking the pan vigorously to coat the pecans well.

• Remove the pan form the heat and stir the pecans. Turn them out of the pan onto the wax paper to cool. Separate them from each other just after placing on the wax paper so that they won't stick together.

Candied Pumpkin Seeds

Ingredients

• 1/2 cup pumpkin seeds (pepitas)

• 1/16 tsp salt

• 1 Tbsp maple syrup

Direction

• Place a sheet of wax paper on the kitchen counter. Place the pumpkin seeds in a non-stick skillet over medium-high heat. Cook, stirring frequently, for about 5 minutes. Watch the seeds closely and as they begin to brown reduce the heat to medium.

• Add the salt. Cook for about one minute more until the seeds are browned.

• Add the maple syrup and let it bubble for about ten seconds shaking the pan vigorously to coat the pumpkin seeds well.

• Remove the pan from the heat and stir the pumpkin seeds. Turn them out of the pan onto the wax paper to cool. Separate them into small clumps just after placing on the wax paper so that they won't stick together.

Crispy Quinoa

Ingredients

• 2 cups water

• 1/2 cup quinoa

• 1/4 tsp. salt

Direction

• Place the water in a small sauce pan over high heat.

• When the water boils, add the quinoa and salt. Reduce the heat to a high simmer.

• Partially cover the pan and cook until the water is almost evaporated. Stir occasionally. When the quinoa is done, turn off the heat and cover.

• After about 5 minutes, remove the quinoa to a large mixing bowl. After it has cooled, spread the quinoa thinly on a cookie sheet.

• Let the quinoa dry on the cookie sheet for 2 hours at room temperature.

• Preheat the oven to 325°F.

• Place the cookie sheet in the oven and toast the quinoa for 30 minutes. About every 7 minutes gently stir the quinoa and re-spread it so that it remains a thin layer.

• Cool on the cookie sheet, then store in a tightly sealed container.

Healthy Deviled Eggs

Ingredients

- 2 quarts water

- 6 large eggs

- 2 Tbsp avocado

- 1 tsp olive oil

- 1/8 tsp salt

- fresh ground black pepper (to taste)

- 1/8 tsp paprika

Direction

- Place the water in a small pan over high heat. When the water is boiling, place the eggs (in the shell) gently in the pan and cook at a boil for three minutes. Turn off the heat and let the eggs stand in the hot water for 12 minutes.

- Remove the eggs from the hot water and add to a bowl of ice water.

- While the eggs are cooling, whisk together the avocado, olive oil, salt, and pepper.

- After the eggs are cooled, peel them and pat dry with a paper towel.

- Slice the eggs in half lengthwise and remove the yolks, placing them in the bowl with the avocado mixture.

- Place the egg whites on a plate and place the plate in the refrigerator.

- Using a fork, mash the egg yolks together with the avocado until smooth.

- Scoop the egg yolk mixture evenly into the egg white halves.

- Chill.

- Sprinkle with paprika before serving.

Olive Dust

Ingredients

- 2 cups medium Kalamata olives

Direction

• Preheat the oven to 250°F.

• Spread the olives on a sheet pan.

• Place the pan in the oven.

• Cook for three hours.

• Remove from the oven and let stand on the counter until cool.

• Place the dried olives in a blender or mini-chopper.

• Pulse until the olives are the consistency of fine gravel.

• Serve.

Bread Machine Gluten Free Pizza Dough

Ingredients

• 2/3 cup warm water

• 4 tsp. honey

• 1 cup garbanzo flour (divided)

- 1/2 cup tapioca flour

- 1/2 cup buckwheat flour

- 1/2 cup millet flour

- 1/2 tsp. salt

- 2 tsp. xanthan gum

- 1 1/2 tsp dry active yeast

Direction

- Place the water in the bread machine pan.

- Add the honey and 3/4 cup of garbanzo flour.

- Add the tapioca flour, buckwheat flour, millet flour, salt, and xanthan gum.

- Sprinkle the yeast over the top of the flour.

- Turn on the machine.

- When the machine is complete, remove the dough and divide into four equal pieces.

• Sprinkle a tablespoon of the remaining garbanzo flour on a cutting board and roll out until it is about 1/8 inch thick and about 8 or 9 inches around.

• Cover the dough that you are not going to use immediately in plastic wrap and chill.

• This crust is best baked on a pizza stone for about 4 to 5 minutes. Remove and turn over. Put your selected pizza toppings on the crisped side and then return to the oven for another 10 minutes or so to bake.

Tapenade

Ingredients

• 6 ounces (about 60) pitted kalamata olives

• 3 Tbsp capers

• 1 Tbsp fresh lemon juice

• 2 Tbsp olive oil

• 1/4 tsp fresh ground black pepper

Direction

• Place olives, capers, lemon juice, olive oil and pepper in a blender or small food chopper and process until smooth.

• Chill.

Gluten Free Whole Grain Pizza Crust

Ingredients

• 1 1/4 cups warm water (105°F to 110°F)

• 2 tsp active dry yeast

• 1 tsp honey

• 3/4 cup tapioca flour

• 1/2 cup buckwheat flour

• 1/4 cup white rice flour

• 1/2 cup brown rice flour

• 1/2 cup millet flour

• 2 tsp xanthan gum

• 1/2 tsp salt

• 1 Tbsp olive oil

Direction

• Place 1/4 cup of warm water in a small dish with the yeast and honey. Stir and let stand for 15 minutes.

• Sift the tapioca, buckwheat, white rice flour, brown rice flour, millet flour, xanthan gum and salt into a large mixing bowl.

• Add the remaining 1 cup water with the olive oil to the dry ingredients. Using a rubber spatula, fold the mixture together until well blended. The dough will not be very smooth.

• Add the yeast and water. Fold together.

• Using your hands, knead the dough with a fold and turn motion. Press down on the dough ball with the heel of your hand until slightly flattened. Fold, turn 90° and repeat until the dough is smooth - about three to five minutes.

• Form the dough into a ball.

• Put about 2 inches of warm water in the bottom of the sink.

• Place the bowl with the dough ball in the sink and cover with a kitchen towel. Let stand for 45 minutes and knead a second time for about two minutes.

• Return the bowl to the sink and let stand for another 45 minutes.

• When ready to bake, place a pizza stone or cookie sheet in the oven and preheat to 450°F.

• Cut the dough into 4 balls and flatten into rounds. Pre-bake for 3 minutes on one side and then turn. Bake for another 2 minutes.

• Top with your selected pizza toppings and then return to the oven for 10 to 15 minutes.

CONCLUSION

A hiatal hernia develops when the stomach protrudes through the diaphragm into the chest cavity. This can lead to a weakening of the LES of the esophagus, resulting in symptoms like heartburn and regurgitation.

Reducing or avoiding foods that relax the LES, such as spicy, acidic, and fried foods, can help alleviate these symptoms. While there isn't a specific diet to follow after hernia repair surgery, you may need to temporarily adhere to a dysphagia diet as swallowing difficulties are common post-surgery.

Modifying your dietary intake may alleviate acid reflux caused by a hiatal hernia. If you're having difficulty identifying your triggers, consider keeping a food diary.

Triggers for acid reflux vary from person to person, so maintaining a food journal and recording any symptoms can be beneficial.

Certain foods that bother one individual may not affect another. Record what you've consumed and how it affects you. Over time, you may notice patterns and identify which foods are causing your symptoms.

9 798323 473243